MOXIBUSTION THERAPY HANDBOOK

Beginners Guide To Healing With Moxibustion, Techniques, Traditions, And Transformations

VICTORY DENNIS

Table of Contents

Introduction 5

CHAPTER ONE..8

Moxibustion: Fundamental Concepts And Ideas 8

Methods Of Moxibustion And Their Varieties...12

CHAPTER TWO 18

The Evidence Supporting Moxibustion.18

Material And Supplies 23

CHAPTER THREE.......................................29

Cautionary Precautions 29

Setting Up The Therapeutic Environment 34

Techniques For Moxibustion 39

CHAPTER FOUR..45

Moxibution Methods...........................45

Acupuncture, Moxibustion, And Traditional Chinese Medicine 50

CHAPTER FIVE 56

Self-Application Methods That Are Safe

....56

Incorporating Moxibustion Into Routine

Activities 63

CHAPTER SIX 68

Important Cautionary Notes And Caveats

....68

Confronting Shared Obstacles 73

The Conclusion 79

THE END 83

Introduction

In moxibustion therapy, a form of traditional Chinese medicine (TCM), specific areas of the body are stimulated by the burning of a desiccated herb known as moxa (made from the leaves of the Artemisia vulgaris plant). It is often used in conjunction with acupuncture.

During moxibustion therapy, a small quantity of moxa is burned near or on acupuncture points or meridians (energy pathways) in the body. The herb is then ignited and burnt at a low temperature to produce a penetrating fire. It is believed that burning moxa promotes healing and balance by increasing the circulation of qi (vital energy) and blood throughout the body.

In TCM, moxibustion therapy is used to alleviate pain, arthritis, digestive issues, menstrual irregularities, and even certain pulmonary diseases. It is also used to enhance general health and strengthen the immune system.

Direct moxibustion is performed by burning a moxa stick or cone over the affected area, whereas indirect moxibustion is performed by burning a moxa cone over the affected area.

Even though moxibustion therapy has a long history of use in traditional Chinese medicine and remains popular among modern practitioners, questions persist regarding its efficacy and safety.

Before beginning treatment, it is advised to consult a medical professional or licensed acupuncturist who is familiar with moxibustion.

CHAPTER ONE
Moxibustion: Fundamental Concepts And Ideas

The foundation of moxibustion therapy is traditional Chinese medicine (TCM). The following are key concepts underlying moxibustion:

• According to TCM, qi (vital energy) flows through a network of meridians (energy conduits) that spans the entire human body. The meridians are nerve, blood vessel, and other tissue networks that regulate the body's processes. Moxibustion's purpose is to restore the natural passage of qi through the meridians.

• In traditional Chinese medicine (TCM), yin and yang are foundational concepts that are sometimes used interchangeably. Yin is associated with darkness, chill, and inactivity, while yang is associated with light, heat, and motion.

• A healthy organism requires a stable balance between yin and yang. It is believed that moxibustion can treat yin and yang imbalances.

• According to TCM, certain diseases are induced by the presence of cold and dampness in the body. When qi and blood cannot circulate freely, discomfort and dysfunction may ensue.

• Cold and dampness are regarded as pathogenic factors that can impede the flow of qi and blood. Moxibustion is frequently used to restore the natural flow of qi and eliminate symptoms of cold and moisture.

• Moxibustion therapy is frequently employed to warm and strengthen localized body portions. The burning of moxa increases circulation, soothes sore muscles, and reduces discomfort. It is believed to restore qi and boost the immune system.

• Similar to acupuncture, moxibustion therapy involves the selective stimulation of acupuncture points and meridian pathways. These acupoints are chosen based on the symptoms of the patient and the desired treatment outcome.

• You can administer moxibustion directly to the skin, indirectly with ginger or salt, or with moxa sticks and cones.

These concepts and ideas provide the foundation for understanding how moxibustion therapy is said to function in traditional Chinese medicine. While these concepts have been handed down for centuries in traditional Chinese medicine, their scientific basis and mechanisms of action are currently under investigation.

Methods Of Moxibustion And Their Varieties

In moxibustion therapy, a variety of approaches are available, all of which are tailored to the individual patient. Typical moxibustion techniques consist of the following:

1. A small cone or ball of moxa is applied directly on the skin at a predetermined acupuncture point.

After lighting the moxa, it should blaze for some time before being extinguished. This method can be used to generate concentrated, localized heat. There are two distinct varieties of this occurrence:

• The warming effect is accomplished without leaving a scar when the moxa cone or ball is removed from the skin before it ignites.

• Direct moxibustion may result in scarring if the moxa cone or ball is left in position long enough to burn the skin, leaving behind a blister or a small scar. Utilization of this method is declining.

2. In order to perform indirect moxibustion, a medium is used to produce a barrier between the moxa and the skin, thereby reducing the intensity of the heat. Ginger, garlic, and sodium are the most commonly used carriers.

Traditionally, moxa is utilized by placing it on top of the medium, lighting it on fire, and allowing it to burn gently. This warms the medium, which in turn warms the epidermis and acupuncture point below.

3. In moxa stick moxibustion, a moxa stick resembling a moxa cigar is utilized. Following the selection of an acupuncture point or location, the moxa stick is ignited and held close to the skin to allow the heat to penetrate the tissue.

By using circular or undulating motions, the therapist disperses the heat from the moxa stick rather than concentrating it in one area. This technique is commonly employed to evenly and gradually heat a larger area.

4. The practice of needle moxibustion combines acupuncture and moxibustion. A moxa cone or ball is attached to the shaft of an acupuncture needle.

Following the selection of an acupuncture site, moxa is ignited and a needle is inserted. The needle transfers the heat from the smoldering moxa to the acupuncture point.

5. Warm needle moxibustion is a variation of needle moxibustion in which a heated needle is used. When an acupuncture needle is implanted into a patient and moxa is burned, both the needle and the acupuncture point are heated.

These are a few of the most common procedures in moxibustion therapy. Diagnosis, treatment objectives, and the practitioner's expertise all play a role in determining the technique employed.

Consult a physician or acupuncturist who specializes in moxibustion to determine which technique is ideal for your particular condition.

CHAPTER TWO

The Evidence Supporting Moxibustion

Modern science is still uncovering the processes underlying moxibustion therapy, so additional research is necessary to adequately explain its effects.

Numerous studies have been conducted on the physiological and biochemical responses to moxibustion, shedding light on its potential mechanisms of action.

Some moxibustion research has produced the following findings:

• The thermal stimulation produced by moxibustion is believed to be a critical factor in its therapeutic benefits.

It has been demonstrated that the heat produced by moxibustion improves circulation, dilates blood vessels, and accelerates metabolism in the targeted area. According to scientific studies, moxibustion increases local skin temperature and microcirculation.

• Another effect of moxibustion is modulation of the immune system. Studies have demonstrated that it stimulates the production of natural killer (NK) cells, a type of immune cell that helps the body fend off infections and tumors.

• Moxibustion has also been shown to influence the release and production of cytokines and neuropeptides, all of which are involved in immunological function.

• Neurotransmitter and neuroendocrine chemical effects of

moxibustion have been scientifically documented. Serotonin, norepinephrine, and beta-endorphin levels have been shown to change as a result of moxibustion therapy. These chemicals have the ability to influence mood, pain perception, and stress responses.

In a variety of research contexts, moxibustion has been shown to have anti-inflammatory and analgesic effects. It inhibits the production of inflammatory mediators and reduces inflammatory markers.

By modulating endogenous pain modulation mechanisms and

influencing pain perception pathways, moxibustion can reduce pain.

• The effects of moxibustion on the autonomic nervous system, which regulates involuntary bodily processes, have been documented. Its ability to moderate sympathetic and parasympathetic processes results in improved homeostasis and equilibrium.

However, additional high-quality research, including well-designed clinical studies, is required to further understand the mechanisms of action and validate the efficacy of moxibustion, as these results only shed light on the possible physiological effects of moxibustion.

If you are considering moxibustion therapy, it is best to consult with a physician or acupuncturist who can tailor their care to your specific requirements.

Material And Supplies

Tools and materials designed specifically for moxibustion therapy are required for effective and secure treatment. The following are frequently employed in moxibustion:

• Moxa is the common name given to the desiccated herb Artemisia vulgaris. This herb is used extensively in moxibustion as its primary fuel source. Moxa can be purchased in numerous forms, including loose moxa, moxa rods, moxa cones, and moxa rolls, to name a few. It is up to the practitioner to determine how and what type of moxa to use.

• A moxa holder is a device used to maintain moxa lit and accessible throughout the treatment. It can be constructed from metal, ceramic, and additional materials.

The purpose of the moxa holder is to prevent the moxa from rolling over or burning the surrounding area while it is being burned.

• Acupuncture Needles Certain types of moxibustion, including needle moxibustion and heated needle moxibustion, employ acupuncture needles. These tiny, sterile, single-use needles are suitable for acupuncture and moxibustion treatments.

• Safety precautions must be taken because moxibustion involves the application of heat and the combustion of materials.

To prevent injury, the practitioner should wear protective mitts, dispose of burnt moxa on a heat-resistant surface or container, and cover the treatment area with a protective sheet or cloth.

• In indirect moxibustion, mediums are inserted between the patient's skin and the burning moxa. Ginger, garlic, and salt are frequently employed as carriers. These insulators reduce the intensity of the heat and prevent the moxa from coming into direct contact with the epidermis.

• A fireproof ashtray or container is necessary for accumulating and burning moxa ashes safely. This eliminates potential fire hazards and provides a central waste disposal facility.

• Alcohol swabs are utilized to remove debris from the treatment region prior to moxibustion. They contribute to a clean and germ-free environment.

• Ignition Tools: There are multiple methods for igniting the moxa, and each requires a distinct set of ignition tools. This category comprises lighters, matches, and candles. To prevent accidents, fire-starting apparatus must be handled with care.

Several instruments and materials may be employed, depending on the moxibustion technique, the practitioner's preferences, and the patient's condition.

Consult a registered acupuncturist or other medical specialist for assistance in deciding which supplies to use for your moxibustion therapy.

CHAPTER THREE
Cautionary Precautions

To safeguard both the practitioner and the patient's health, moxibustion therapy must be administered with extreme care. Important precautions include the following:

• Since moxibustion involves the use of combustible materials, it is essential to take appropriate fire precautions. Moxibustion should be performed in a well-ventilated area, away from anything flammable.

As a precaution, keep a fire blanket or extinguisher on site. After each use, the moxa must be completely extinguished before being placed in a fireproof container.

• It is essential to protect the patient's epidermis from the heat produced when moxa is burned. Use a towel or heat-resistant pad as a barrier if you do not want the moxa to contact your skin. This reduces the likelihood of injury or distress.

Maintain open channels of communication with the patient throughout the duration of therapy to ensure that they are feeling well and receiving the necessary care. Inquire whether they are experiencing any discomfort. It is essential to address any concerns or unease immediately, which promotes open communication.

• Inquire if the patient has any known allergies or sensitivities, particularly to moxa or other treatment-related substances. Avoid moxibustion if the patient has an allergy to mugwort or related flora.

• When working with acupuncture needles, moxa, and any other instruments, observe strict standards of hygiene and sterility. When performing needle moxibustion, it is essential to use sterile, disposable needles and maintain the cleanliness of all instruments and surfaces.

• Protect yourself from burns by observing these precautions as a practitioner. Gloves should be worn when directly applying moxibustion techniques. Handle moxa and other burning substances with caution to prevent skin contact.

• When selecting patients, it is essential to ascertain whether moxibustion therapy is an appropriate treatment. Consider the individual's age, gender, general health, any potential hazards, and individual preferences.

Pregnant women, individuals with certain skin conditions, and those who are extremely heat sensitive may not be ideal candidates for moxibustion.

• Ensure your qualifications to practice moxibustion by completing a training program and obtaining certification. Consult a physician or licensed acupuncturist for guidance on how to safely and effectively perform the technique.

These precautions are intended to serve as guidelines. It is essential to consult with a competent healthcare professional or licensed acupuncturist in order to receive specific safety instructions and recommendations.

Setting Up The Therapeutic
Environment

The treatment space for moxibustion must be meticulously prepared to ensure the patient's safety, comfort, and optimal conditions for healing. Consider the following details as you prepare the treatment area:

• Preserve a pristine environment for your therapy sessions. Remove any obstacles to movement or potential hazards you discover.

• Because smoldering moxa produces smoke and a pungent odor, moxibustion therapy requires adequate ventilation. Open windows or switch on the fans to keep the air circulating and the room feeling fresh.

• The treatment area must have sufficient illumination for the procedure. The therapy can be performed more precisely and safely in a well-lit area. Calm the anxieties with a soft, diffused light source.

• Furniture: Ensure that the patient has a comfortable place to lie down or unwind for the duration of the session, such as a treatment table or reclining chair.

In order for patients to feel at ease while receiving care, it is essential that treatment areas contain clean, stable, and comfortable furniture.

• Protect the right to anonymity of patients by creating a treatment location away from the main lobby or waiting area. By separating participants with draperies, screens, or partitions, you can create a more intimate environment.

• The temperature in the treatment chamber should be maintained at a level that does not cause patients discomfort.

• Due to the use of heat in moxibustion therapy, it is crucial that the room temperature be agreeable.

Consider installing variable-setting climate control systems to maintain a comfortable environment.

• Use soft music, the sounds of nature, or other calming sounds to create a tranquil atmosphere. If it is safe to do so, attempt aromatherapy with lavender or chamomile essential oils to help the patient relax.

• Prepare for Emergencies Keep fire extinguishers and fire blankets accessible in the event of an emergency. You should know where everything is located and how to use the available instruments.

• Keep your moxa, needles, and other instruments in an organized space. To avoid complications or delays in treatment, keep them organized and easily accessible.

• Provide a place where the patient can speak freely and without interruption. Before, during, and after therapy, allow the patient to voice their opinions and concerns in a comfortable setting.

Always consider the patient's specific needs and preferences when designing the therapy environment. Moxibustion therapy requires a clean, comfortable, and secure environment; therefore, it is essential to regularly evaluate and make any necessary adjustments.

Techniques For Moxibustion

Moxibustion is a form of traditional Chinese medicine in which the herb moxa (dried Artemisia vulgaris) is incinerated over acupuncture points or other body areas to promote healing.

Moxibustion therapy employs various techniques, each with its own advantages and disadvantages. Typical moxibustion applications are as follows:

1. In direct moxibustion, a small cone or pellet of moxa is placed directly onto the skin at the targeted acupuncture point. The moxa is ignited and incinerated slowly and steadily until extinguished or removed. Two distinct types of direct moxibustion exist:

• Direct moxibustion, also referred to as moxacone or moxaball therapy, is a form of acupuncture that provides a warming sensation without leaving a wound on the skin because the moxa is removed before it burns.

• If the moxa cone or ball is left on the skin long enough to burn it and leave a blister or scar, direct moxibustion can induce scarring. Utilization of this method is declining.

2. Indirect moxibustion involves using ginger, garlic, or salt slices as a barrier between the burning moxa and the epidermis. Traditionally, moxa is utilized by placing it on top of the medium, lighting it on fire, and allowing it to burn gently. This warms the medium, which in turn warms the epidermis and acupuncture point below. Due to its gentler and more controlled application of heat, indirect moxibustion is a common treatment.

3. Moxa used in moxa stick moxibustion is rolled into a cigar shape and set on a moxa stick. Following the selection of an acupuncture point or location, the moxa stick is ignited and held close to the skin to allow the heat to penetrate the tissue.

The therapist may wave or rotate the moxa stick to disperse the heat equitably and prevent burns. Frequently, moxibustion with a moxa stick is utilized to administer gentle and uniform heat to a larger area.

4. The practice of needle moxibustion combines acupuncture and moxibustion. A moxa cone or ball is attached to the shaft of an acupuncture needle. Following the selection of an acupuncture site, moxa is ignited and a needle is inserted.

The needle transfers the heat from the smoldering moxa to the acupuncture point. Utilizing a needle for moxibustion enables for the precise application of heat.

5. Warm needle moxibustion is a variation of needle moxibustion in which a heated needle is used. When an acupuncture needle is implanted into a patient and moxa is burned, both the needle and the acupuncture point are heated.

In warm needle moxibustion, acupuncture and moxibustion are combined for therapeutic purposes.

These are some of the most common moxibustion applications. The choice of technique is influenced by the patient's condition, the intended therapeutic outcome, and the practitioner's level of education and experience.

A skilled acupuncturist or other medical professional can assist you in determining which moxibustion technique will be most beneficial for your condition.

CHAPTER FOUR
Moxibution Methods

Traditional Chinese medicine remedies, such as moxibustion, are effective for a wide range of diseases and symptoms. Typically, moxibustion is used for the following:

• Moxibustion is frequently used to alleviate pain, particularly musculoskeletal discomfort, joint pain, and menstrual cramping. By increasing blood flow, relaxing muscles, and decreasing inflammation, moxibustion can reduce pain.

• Indigestion, diarrhea, and abdominal pain are among the digestive conditions that moxibustion has been shown to alleviate. Moxibustion is utilized to regulate gastrointestinal function and improve digestion by stimulating specific acupuncture points associated with the gastrointestinal tract.

• Moxibustion has been utilized to enhance health and well-being by strengthening the immune system. It has the potential to strengthen the immune system, reduce susceptibility to illness, and aid in the healing of the body.

• Moxibustion is frequently employed to treat respiratory conditions such as asthma, chronic bronchitis, and wheezing. Stimulating specific points on the body, moxibustion works to relax the respiratory muscles, reduce inflammation, and open the airways.

• Moxibustion is frequently utilized to treat menstrual disorders, including agonizing or irregular periods. It can alleviate menstrual pain, enhance blood flow to the pelvic region, and normalize hormone levels.

• Moxibustion can improve fertility and reproductive health in general. Moxibustion can enhance reproductive health by increasing blood flow to the reproductive organs, restoring hormonal balance, and decreasing inflammation.

• Moxibustion can be administered prior to the onset of a cold, virus, or respiratory infection to enhance the immune system's ability to combat illness. It may strengthen the immune system and increase the body's resistance to microbes that cause disease.

• Moxibustion is sometimes used to restore harmony to the mind and spirit by treating conditions such as tension, anxiety, and depression.

Moxibustion is a technique used in traditional Chinese medicine to alleviate tension, improve mood, and restore physical and emotional balance by stimulating acupuncture points.

Depending on the patient's symptoms, moxibustion can be administered in a variety of methods, and the treatment should be modified accordingly.

Medical and acupuncture professionals are best adapted to administer moxibustion because they can evaluate your health and determine the most effective treatment.

Acupuncture, Moxibustion, And Traditional Chinese Medicine

Moxibustion is frequently employed in conjunction with acupuncture and other Traditional Chinese Medicine (TCM) techniques.

When these techniques are combined, therapeutic effects can be amplified and a more holistic approach to health and wellness can be provided. Combining moxibustion with acupuncture and TCM has the following appearance:

• Traditional Chinese Medicine (TCM) incorporates both acupuncture and moxibustion. When conducting acupuncture, fine needles are inserted into specific acupuncture points on the body, whereas moxibustion involves the burning of moxa near or on the acupuncture points.

By combining these techniques, the outcomes of each can be amplified.

For example, acupuncture can be used to stimulate acupuncture points and regulate the flow of Qi (energy) in the body, whereas moxibustion can provide additional thermal therapy to augment the effect of acupuncture and improve blood circulation.

• Moxibustion is a prevalent treatment in traditional Chinese medicine and is founded on TCM diagnostic principles. Traditional Chinese Medicine (TCM) practitioners determine the optimal acupuncture points and moxibustion techniques by analyzing a patient's overall constitution, patterns of disharmony, and symptoms.

When combined with acupuncture, moxibustion can provide a highly individualized treatment plan for treating the underlying imbalances revealed by TCM diagnosis.

• Moxibustion can be used to either tonify or distribute the body's Qi and circulation. In TCM theory, tonification means to strengthen and nourish the body's Qi and blood, whereas dispersion means to stimulate the flow and evacuation of Qi and blood that have become excessive or indolent.

Depending on the patient's condition, moxibustion can be used to intensify the effects of tonifying or dispersing specific acupuncture points.

• Acupuncture and moxibustion rely on an understanding of the meridian (energy) channels of the body and the relationship between acupuncture points and organ systems.

TCM theory relates each acupuncture point to a specific body part and meridian. When acupuncture is combined with moxibustion, the practitioner is able to target specific meridians and organs, restoring health and preventing disease.

• Acupuncture, moxibustion, and other TCM treatments such as herbal medicine, food therapy, and lifestyle recommendations can be incorporated into a singular holistic treatment plan, also known as a "integrative treatment approach."

By addressing the underlying imbalances that have contributed to health problems, these modalities support the body's inherent capacity for self-healing.

The best method to determine if acupuncture, moxibustion, or any other TCM modality is appropriate for you is to schedule an appointment with a TCM-trained healthcare professional or acupuncturist.

CHAPTER FIVE
Self-Application Methods That Are Safe

However, there are a number of safe self-application techniques that can be used with caution in the absence of a qualified healthcare professional or licensed acupuncturist. Several examples are as follows:

1. Moxa Stick on an Acupuncture Point:

• Select an acupuncture point to activate if you wish to stimulate one. Consult a trustworthy acupuncture reference book or an experienced acupuncturist for assistance when selecting acupuncture sites.

• Maintain the moxa stick two to three centimeters away from the target area.

• Light the moxa stick's end on fire and maintain a safe distance from the skin.

• For 5 to 10 minutes, or until you feel a faint warmth, move the moxa stick around the affected area in a circular or wavy pattern.

• Keep the moxa stick away from flammable materials, including your epidermis.

2. Utilization of a Moxa Box for Remote Moxibustion:

• Moxa should be preserved in a ceramic bowl or a dedicated container.

• Once the moxa has been ignited, allow it to continue burning until a constant heat is produced.

• Stimulating acupuncture points and other areas is possible by holding the moxa box at a safe distance from them.

• Move the moxa box in a circular or wavy motion for 5 to 10 minutes, or until you feel a mild warmth, while maintaining a safe distance from the skin.

• Prevent potential injuries and flames by securely anchoring the moxa box.

3. Moxa vegetation:

• Acquire some moxa self-application patches. These patches typically contain compressed moxa and come in a variety of standard shapes.

• To apply moxa patches safely and effectively, you must follow the instructions included with the patches. Typically, the patches are applied directly to the targeted acupuncture point.

• Light the moxa and allow it to burn for the allotted amount of time.

• Keep the moxa patch away from anything that could cause a fire or injury.

• Self-application of moxibustion is not risk-free; therefore, it is essential to take precautions and follow standard safety procedures. Consider the following safety precautions:

• Acquaint yourself with the techniques by learning them from a trained medical professional or licensed acupuncturist.

• Learn about any associated risks or contraindications with specific acupuncture points or health conditions.

• Never leave smoldering moxa unattended; always carry a fire blanket or fire extinguisher.

• Always use moxibustion in a well-ventilated area away from any ignition sources.

• Begin with brief sessions at lower temperatures in order to determine your tolerance and response.

• Stop the session if you experience pain, discomfort, or any other adverse effects.

Always consult with a competent healthcare practitioner or licensed acupuncturist for individualized advice and safe administration of moxibustion procedures. The advice you receive will be tailored to your particular health situation and needs.

Incorporating Moxibustion Into Routine Activities

Regularly incorporating moxibustion into your self-care routine can have numerous beneficial effects. Following are some practical applications of moxibustion.

• Incorporate moxibustion into your daily or nightly regimen at the same time each day or night. Now is the time to relax and consider what is best for your physical and mental health. Choose a tranquil location where you won't disturb anyone while performing moxibustion.

• If you are a regular practitioner of meditation or mindfulness, moxibustion could be an excellent addition to your session. Before or after your meditation session, choose an acupuncture point or location to administer moxibustion. The therapeutic heat of moxibustion can deepen your meditation practice.

• Throughout the day, take brief breaks to focus on self-care. Take advantage of these lulls to administer a brief moxibustion treatment to an acupuncture point. It can assist in calming nerves, reducing tension, and enhancing concentration and work output.

• If you already participate in a regular exercise regimen, moxibustion could be a beneficial addition either before or after your workout. By increasing blood circulation and body temperature, moxibustion facilitates post-exercise recovery and accelerates the healing process. Select the acupuncture points that will benefit your exercise regimen the most.

• Incorporate moxibustion into your nightly regimen to help you relax and get a better night's rest. Try Yin Tang (the space between your eyebrows) or Shen Men (the tip of your ear) moxibustion before bed to relax your mind and body.

The cozy environment can help you unwind and get a decent night's sleep.

When incorporating moxibustion into your daily routine, always prioritize safety and employ proper technique. Visiting a physician or licensed acupuncturist is a good idea if you want to choose the correct points and perform moxibustion safety.

It is also important to note that moxibustion is not suitable for everyone or every health concern. Before incorporating moxibustion into your daily routine, you should discuss any preexisting medical conditions or concerns with your physician.

CHAPTER SIX
Important Cautionary Notes And Caveats

Moxibustion has the potential to be an effective treatment, but there are a number of precautions and limitations to consider. These details will assist you in performing moxibustion correctly and safely. Listed below are some exceptions and warnings.

• Some individuals may have sensitivities or hypersensitivity to moxa or its smoke. Please refrain from using moxibustion if you have ever experienced a negative reaction to Artemisia vulgaris (the plant used in the practice). If you are interested in alternative treatments, you should consult a physician first.

• Extremely heat-sensitive individuals may find moxibustion unbearable or excruciating. If you've never tried moxibustion before, it's essential to begin with shorter sessions and less intense heat.

• Avoid using moxibustion on a specific area of skin if there are open lesions, rashes, burns, or other skin issues. Due to the high temperatures it generates, moxibustion can exacerbate these symptoms or cause additional irritation. The use of moxibustion should be delayed until the skin has completely recovered.

• Moxibustion has a long history of use during pregnancy, including for breech infant flip. However, the treatment should only be administered by a trained medical professional with expertise in prenatal care and moxibustion during pregnancy.

As there are acupuncture locations and techniques that should be avoided during pregnancy, it is vital to seek the advice of an experienced practitioner.

• Individuals with cancer or tumors should exercise prudence when using moxibustion. Before deciding whether moxibustion is appropriate for you, consult a physician who is knowledgeable in both cancer and Traditional Chinese Medicine (TCM).

• Patients with a fever or acute inflammation should not undergo moxibustion therapy. Moxibustion, which entails the use of heat, may exacerbate the situation. Do not employ moxibustion until the fever has subsided and the acute irritation has subsided.

• Before attempting moxibustion, if you are taking any medications or have any preexisting medical conditions, you should consult your doctor. Moxibustion may have contraindications or require modification when used in conjunction with specific medical conditions or medications.

Before attempting moxibustion, if you have any preexisting health conditions or concerns, you should consult your doctor or an acupuncturist. They are trained to assess your condition, recommend the most effective treatment, and ensure that moxibustion meets your specific objectives.

Confronting Shared Obstacles

When attempting to incorporate moxibustion into their daily existence, individuals commonly face a number of obstacles. Here are some strategies for handling them:

• Moxibustion is not appropriate for everyone because it produces vapor and has a distinct odor. This issue can be mitigated by opening windows or using a fan to circulate air in the treatment area.

A nearby small fan or air purifier may also help reduce residual smoke and odor. Additionally, it may be advantageous to choose odorless or low-smoke moxa varieties.

• Since moxibustion involves the use of flame, it is vital to take precautions to prevent a fire. Always exercise caution and observe security measures.

Moxibustion should be performed away from anything flammable, and a fire blanket or extinguisher should be available in case of emergency. Ensure that the moxa stick or moxa case is secure so that it does not topple and cause burns.

• Since moxibustion generates heat, it is necessary to regulate the temperature to avoid suffering or burns. When beginning moxibustion, it is advisable to begin with shorter sessions and less intense heat. As you grow accustomed to the sensation, you can extend the duration and increase the temperature. Observe how your body reacts and make adjustments as necessary.

• For moxibustion to be effective, the practitioner must be able to identify and treat specific acupuncture points.

Consult a medical professional or licensed acupuncturist if you have any questions about the appropriate acupuncture points or techniques. They can demonstrate how to perform the exercise and ensure that you're targeting the appropriate areas based on your condition.

• Consistency and self-control are necessary for incorporating moxibustion into one's daily existence. Schedule it, or incorporate it into your daily routine if you meditate or take other self-care breaks. The positive effects of moxibustion can be amplified by incorporating it into one's routine.

• Individual Preference: Moxibustion can be administered for as long or as little time as the patient desires. Try a variety of approaches until you discover one that meets your requirements.

Those who are sensitive to heat may find indirect moxibustion techniques, such as a moxa box or patches, more tolerable. Moxibustion can be administered from a distance and for as long as the patient desires.

• If you are experiencing difficulties or have specific health concerns, you should consult a registered acupuncturist or other medical professional. They can tailor their instructions to your unique requirements and concerns, as well as check in to ensure that you are using moxibustion correctly.

Follow your body's cues and adjust your moxibustion routine accordingly. Stop the session and consult a physician if you continue to experience pain, discomfort, or other adverse effects. They can provide advice tailored to your specific situation.

The Conclusion

Moxibustion is an ancient Chinese medical technique that dates back millennia. Moxa is an Artemisia vulgaris-derived herb that is incinerated to stimulate acupuncture points. In conjunction with acupuncture and other Traditional Chinese Medicine procedures, moxibustion is used to promote health and wellness.

By learning its concepts, techniques, and applications, individuals can benefit from incorporating moxibustion into their self-care practices.

Self-application of moxibustion is safe if the patient takes the necessary precautions, creates a suitable treatment environment, and follows the proper procedures.

There are numerous benefits to incorporating moxibustion into your daily routine, be it a morning or evening ritual, a meditation session, a self-care break, or even before or after exercise.

Nonetheless, certain exceptions and precautions must be taken into account. Moxa can induce reactions in some individuals, and those who are allergic to it, pregnant, or taking certain medications should use it with caution.

To ensure that you are using moxibustion correctly and safely, you must consult a physician or licensed acupuncturist.

Individuals can surmount potential obstacles and maximize their moxibustion practice by addressing concerns such as smoke and odor, fire safety, heat intensity, point position, consistency, personal comfort, and professional supervision.

Including self-care activities such as moxibustion in your wellness regimen can be advantageous, but you should do so with awareness, caution, and consideration for your unique health conditions and preferences.

THE END